Table of Contents

Causes of Bladder Cancer in Females

1. Introduction to Bladder Cancer

The reasons for bladder cancer are complex and multifaceted. Smoking causes nearly 50% of male and female cancers, one of which is non-epidemic. In such cases, the patient suffers family difficulties or has no history of exposure unless the patient personally uses smoke. Despite the continuing development of medicine, the proportion of non-smokers has risen considerably in the last few years. This will explain the research into the non-smoking pathophysiology of bladder cancer, which is undoubtedly increasing.

Bladder cancer is uncontrollable cell growth in the urinary bladder lining, which spreads into the urinary tract. It generally occurs 3-4 times more often in men than in women. According to American statistics, 5-6% of cancers are bladder cancers. Almost 3% are deaths related to bladder cancer. It ranks second in the urinary tract of women. People over 55 are mainly affected, and the average diagnosis is 73 years old. However, the onset occurs in average age groups of 73 and 78 years, respectively. The average age types of males and females are 60 and 63 years. Bladder cancer can recur and is typically curable for early-stage patients, stage 3 or later. If not cured for personal cancer patients, the past will be between 40 and 85 percent.

2. Epidemiology of Bladder Cancer in Females

At the state level, there are six states with an age-adjusted incidence rate ≥12.0 in white women. The remaining states range from 9.0 to <11.9 [upstate: Florida (12.2) and Hawaii (13.2)]. The average age of female bladder cancer patients is approximately 72 years. The reasons for the relatively low incidence in women are not entirely clear, but a number of epidemiologic studies initiated during the 1980s shed some light on its determinants. We concluded from the available data that many protectants are operative in females. Females have only a fraction of the cigarette smoking rate found in men, the principal cause of bladder cancer. Prolonged cigarette smoking is the most significant primary etiological factor for the development of bladder cancer. There is much lower exposure to recognized occupational hazards, and women were much slower to enter these highly at-risk occupations. In addition, the lack of smoking status alone subtracts only a minority of the total variance in men. Smoker women have a 50% higher risk of developing bladder cancer compared with non-smokers, so there are some other unconsidered factors in the general population.

Epidemiology of bladder cancer in females: Incidence is the time rate of the new events. In this scenario, it is the determination of all women who were diagnosed with bladder cancer in a given period in a defined population. Incidence and distribution of such cases vary largely with the country's development, societies, its culture, race, age, urban location, etc. But mostly, the overall incidence in adult women is significantly lower compared with men and represents from 20 to 30% of the men's incidence.

3. Risk Factors for Bladder Cancer in Females

Exposure to cigarette smoke, the main known risk factor common to both men and women, accounts for only part of this risk. Despite lower levels of indoor and outdoor environmental pollution, lung cancer rates in females have been rising, arguing for other factors in the etiology such as hormonal, reproductive, genetic, and also behavioral factors. Bladder candidate risk factors have only been investigated in females, but not in males. There is some evidence for gender differences in the prevalence of some other risk factors for bladder cancer, with, for example, a higher prevalence of urinary infections in women than men, and an increased protective effect of some features of a healthy vaginal flora in women compared with men. Infection and sexual behavior in women should be dynamically evaluated if evidence of gender differences as a cause of bladder cancer or for the differing sexual incubation period between males and women.

Males are at a 3-4 times higher risk of developing bladder cancer than females, but the proportion of bladder cancers that are invasive and lead to death are similar between the sexes in places where smoking is common. It is now almost 30 years since Doll and Hill discussed whether lung cancer in women can be explained by the same causes as in men and posed the question "Bladder cancer in females - when does gender matter?" The ultimate question is "to what extent is the etiology of lung cancer in women distinctive or are gender and disease parallel owners?" via Human knowledge we now know. If gender differences in the natural history of bladder cancer can be explained more as an artifact of lack of exposure to risk factors particular to males rather than by distinct pathologic processes, this could have practical implications.

C. Transitional cell carcinoma - The most prevalent of the three, they should start in the epithelial lining and infiltrate the others. In minimizing the chances of acquiring bladder cancer, the best advice to protect a non-smoking female who is exposed to second-hand smoke must be non-exposed to second-hand smoke.

B. Chronic Tobacco Smoking - Causes urinary bladder carcinoma from the epithelial lining, stroma, and detrusor. In medium risk, an irritated bladder can cause squamous metaplasia. A moderate-grade carcinoma rises and damages the stroma. In some cases, one corner of the epithelial lining breaks and carcinoma sets in. In the low risk, carcinomas arise from transitional epithelium. 10 The predominate tumor can be classified as carcinomas of the bladder, prostatic urethra, ureter, and in female bladder at the papillae and apex.

A. Fulminant Squamous cell carcinoma - Disrupt the internal lining with squamous metaplasia and progresses on disastrous linings, usually the bladder finally falls into carcinoma.

Tobacco smoking has an unfavorable effect on female urinary bladders, some of which are as follows:

Bladder cancer is very closely associated with tobacco smoking. It has been estimated that almost half of urinary bladder cancer cases are tobacco-smoking related. The risk of developing bladder carcinoma is 2 to 3 times higher in women who are tobacco smokers compared to those who do not smoke tobacco. Heavy smokers are 4 to 6 times more at risk. A major portion of the urine, which is drained by the kidneys from the blood, is directed to the urinary bladder. When tobacco is smoked, harmful substances contained in tobacco get mixed with the smoke. The harmful components, like nicotine and tar, get transformed into wasteful matter and excreted out of the body in the urine. In the process, the harmful substances damage the three structures of the urinary bladder: the epithelial lining, the stroma, and the detrusor. The severity of damage of these structures depends on the quantity and duration of tobacco smoked. It has been observed that in a non-smoking environment, many precursors and harmful substances tend to get washed in micturition.

3.2. Occupational Exposures

Working as a hairdresser has a direct impact on human health. Many of the chemicals included in the hairdressing products have potentially harmful effects, which are found regularly in urine. Hormone-related cancers such as bladder cancer are associated with women working in these jobs, but no associations have been found among men. For example, repetitive exposure to 4,4-methylene bis (2-chloroaniline) or combined exposure to 4,4-methylene bis (2-chloroaniline) and 2,4-diaminotoluene seem to increase the risk of bladder cancer in exposed women but have no influence on exposed men.

Exposures to aromatic nitro-, amino- or azo-compounds were also likely in the textile industry and dyeing plants. Female workers were also exposed to occupational agents in the pharmaceutical and metal-mechanic industry or woodworking facilities, given that some studies have reported a higher risk associated with working as a machine operator. Female workers in these jobs were exposed to chemicals that were classified as probable in IARC-carcinogenicity or carcinogenic to laboratory animals and were previously members working as paint manufacturers. Furthermore, occupational agents have been classified as S2 (substances with limited evidence of carcinogenicity), S3 (substances with limited evidence of carcinogenicity), or are not classified for human carcinogenicity.

Only a few studies have specifically investigated whether some occupational exposures are more common in women than in men. Workplace exposure to aromatic amines significantly increases the risk of bladder cancer, but because exposures to these agents among women are very unusual, the impact of these exposures could be significantly lower in women. Exposure to aromatic amines occurs mainly in the rubber, chemical, and metallurgical industries. Jobs in the metal industry that may be associated with occupational exposure to aromatic amines were whether there was a greater risk of female development than male, especially with the equality of exposure and duration of employment.

3.3. Chronic Bladder Inflammation

Having a bladder catheter which is left in for a long time might be a way in which chronic bladder irritation could be caused. There is also evidence that repeated urinary infections or using a urinary catheter for a long time might be associated with some types of bladder cancer. However, much more research is needed to understand the various ways that chronic inflammation may be related to bladder cancer risk. Every time the body has an infection or repairs damaged cells, there is a chance that mistakes will be made when the cells multiply and a cancer may develop. Some studies suggest that daily low-dose antibiotics or estrogen hormone replacement therapy in women might reduce the risk of long-term bladder inflammation, and some doctors and nurses may suggest using estrogen cream if you find that you get lots of bladder infections after menopause.

Inflammation is a natural bodily response to irritants or injury and is often part of the normal healing process. Sometimes, though, inflammation can be longer-lasting or ongoing. Chronic inflammation is thought to cause changes in cells that might make them more likely to become cancers. Chronic bladder infections by a parasite called Schistosoma haematobium can, after many years, lead to bladder cancer. Bladder infections (cystitis) caused by other types of bacteria are common, but they do not seem to increase bladder cancer risk. Conditions that can cause chronic bladder inflammation, such as long-term bladder catheters and some more rare problems with the way the bladder develops, increase the risk of squamous cell

carcinoma (SCC) of the bladder, the second most common
type.

4. Genetic and Hereditary Factors

2. Currently, the specific genetic factors that confer a heightened risk of urothelial bladder cancer remain uncertain for just one condition known as hereditary non-polyposis colorectal cancer. This is characterized by a loss-of-function mutation in the DNA mismatch repair genes that include MLH1, MSH2, MSH6, and PMS2. The estimated lifetime risk of female relatives (daughters and sisters) of these patients developing bladder cancer stands at around 10 percent. Further research may discover additional genetic factors attributed to a higher incidence of urothelial bladder cancer risks in females, but none have been conclusively identified at present. Inherited genetic mutations that predispose women to a greater likelihood of developing kidney cancer are also probably associated with an increased risk of bladder cancer in women. These hereditary conditions are considered throughout the management of people who have developed renal cancer.

1. If bladder cancer, especially urothelial bladder cancer, is found in close family members of a female, it may increase her likelihood of getting the disease. The regular lining of the bladder is a surface known as the urothelial cells, and cancer arising from this tissue or cell type is known as urothelial bladder cancer. Nonetheless, this cause accounts for only a small proportion of the conditions that give rise to bladder cancer.

5. Hormonal Influences on Bladder Cancer Risk

If females are a more frequent study population in research on the influence of hormonal factors on the chronic occurrence of urinary incontinence and the role of these factors in the development of overactive lower urinary tract syndrome (OAB) and interstitial cystitis/bladder pain syndrome (IC/BPS), this is due to greater complexity urogenital neurotransmitter biology and a system that integrates local (in the pelvis) and general (organism) control of the bladder function of the brain-bladder axis. Trauma to the central nervous system (CNS) and/or peripheral nervous system (PNS) with a transition to the subcortical system and/or cortical centers can result from a car accident with injuries to the lumbar and pelvic spine, or from an intracranial accident. Long-term estradiol treatment in elderly women increases the frequency of schizophrenia and stroke and 2% per annum (for medium age = 74 years) increases the incidence of dementia. Progestogen alone, which suppresses the action of estrogen – strong carcinogens, only affects balanced mood, which is important for the pathology of the bladder and leads to a 30% increase in the risk of breast cancer during pregnancy. Hormonal factors influence the pathophysiology of OAB and IC/BPS by altering the function of M and F neurotransmitters. The sudden cessation of estradiol production in vitro leads to overactive bladder syndrome (BVF) in postmenopausal women. The clinical course of urinary incontinence is strictly associated with the differentiation of urothelial cells in organ anatomopathological examination.

Sexual dimorphism in the incidence and etiology of urothelial bladder cancer in females still lacks a clear scientific explanation. The role of hormonal factors in the development of terminal cell kidney cancer and squamous cell vulvar cancer is based on well-established scientific evidence. Acute or overall estrogen deficiency is a factor affecting the decline of urinary system function (kidney, ureters, bladder, urethra) in the elderly and women during menopause. The decrease in bladder function intensifies vaginal atrophy, which can lead to secondary, more frequent bacterial infections of the bladder, urethra, and kidneys. The article presents issues in the field of research related to the role of independent hormonal factors in the carcinogenic transformation process (initiating, promoting, progression) of urothelium in men and women, according to IKNLM/WHO classification. In order to better understand the etiopathogenesis of urothelial lesions leading to bladder cancer, risk factors related to the patient's sexual orientation and hormonal status should be analyzed in more detail. They also influence changes in the biological properties of bladder cancer, such as cell differentiation, degree of invasiveness - staging, and the degree of neovascularization of the neoplasm. The article was developed on the basis of the available literature data and original work.

6. Dietary Factors and Lifestyle Choices

In women only, the low intake of fried foods has gone on to prove an association with a lowered risk of relapse in non-muscle invasive bladder cancer. The outcome of interest in any such study is the association of dietary and lifestyle factors with the outcomes (relapse, progression, death). Genitourinary cancer variables may confound the urinary bladder adenocarcinoma variables of interest. Thus, the study of dietary and lifestyle factors with standardly measured variables compares KLH, an amino acid, with relapse and death in urinary bladder cancer patients.

While diet has not been examined as a risk factor for female bladder cancer, the intake of fruits, vegetables, legumes, and fiber have all been studied in the context of bladder cancer survival and recurrence. Interestingly, apple intake has been associated with a reduced risk of total recurrent or relapsed bladder cancer in men and women. While "apple intake" itself is not an established variable, the value - defined as anything greater than 8.1 mg of apple intake - is proven to reduce relapse or recurrence in non-muscle-invasive patients.

Smoking is a clear risk factor for bladder cancer in women, and women who smoke carry a higher risk than men. Obesity in women is a protective factor against bladder cancer, and obese individuals carry a reduced risk. Thus, overweight women may have reduced bladder cancer risk. A normal BMI carried a reduced risk of bladder cancer compared to an overweight BMI in women.

There are dietary and lifestyle elements that have been proven to increase and decrease the risk of bladder cancer in women. Sedentary behavior has been shown to increase the risk of bladder cancer overall. Furthermore, sedentary individuals have a bladder cancer risk that is increased by 6%. As such, women who engage in sedentary time may have a higher risk of bladder cancer, though more work is needed.

6.1. Diet High in Processed Meats

Processed meats contain cancer-causing nitrate and nitrite preservatives, as well as natural compounds called amines. Together, these form powerful carcinogens, called nitrosamines, in the body, and one type in particular, NIN, was recently linked to colon cancer in animal studies. A diet high in fruits and vegetables, however, was found to lower women's risk of developing bladder cancer, which is consistent with previous research. Fruits and vegetables contain powerful antioxidants and other healthful compounds that lower the risk of other types of cancer as well. In particular, women who ate at least 10 servings of fruits and vegetables per day had a 65 percent reduction in their risk of developing the disease. The link between a diet high in fruits and vegetables and a reduced risk of bladder cancer was stronger in women who ate at least one serving of processed meats every day. Thus, women who eat a healthful diet that includes fruits and vegetables can still benefit from kicking the processed-meat habit.

Bladder cancer is the fifth most common cancer in the United States today. Smoking is the leading cause of this disease, but dietary factors may explain some cases of bladder cancer in females. Gertig and colleagues conducted a study on women in western New York that showed a substantial link between consuming processed meats - including bacon, ham, and hot dogs - and an elevated risk of this form of cancer. Women who ate at least one serving of a type of processed meat per day were more than three times as likely to develop bladder cancer than women who never ate it.

6.2. Low Fluid Intake

There is no consensus among doctors and nutritionists about the rate of drinking water. Serious discussion still exists on who is correct. One of the initial reactions may lead to an inconsistent level of trust from one side towards others' advice. Water is the primary foodstuff. We breathe, fight, improve, and consume. It acts as a solvent and carries out bodily functions including digestion, intake of vitamins and nutrients, and regulation of temperature. Participation by body fluids is up to 90%. Approximately 60% is occupied by water in an adult man, 55% in an adult female. Long sleep overnight has traditionally been fasting, and "breakfast" is to consume a solid meal. Water has not been addressed previously in nutrition studies.

Low fluid intake can increase the risk of bladder cancer in females as the toxins are not flushed from the system, and they remain accumulating in the bladder. Studies have shown that daily intake of water (at least 8 to 9 glasses) may help decrease the risk of bladder cancer as toxins in the bladder are diluted and washed away. The bladder might become prone to irritation or even carcinogens when a person is not hydrated enough. Monitoring the color of urine may help determine if more water is needed. The urine usually should have a pale yellow color to signal sufficient hydration. When the organ that stores urine, the bladder, is not functioning correctly, nutrients and waste are more concentrated because the amount of water expelled as urine can be decreased. This raises the chance of cells in the bladder being exposed to toxic effects.

Moreover, when urine is too concentrated, natural waste may cause irritation and damage to the tissue of the cells lining the bladder. This may elevate the risk of developing bladder cancer.

6.3. Physical Inactivity

The main file includes a subfile in electronic literature called 6.3 Physical Inactivity. This subfile, written by our Indian collaborator Ramakrishnan S., contains electronic text that discusses physical inactivity as a potential cause of cancer. This information focuses on damage to health that physical inactivity can cause, such as heart disease, diabetes, stroke, and obesity. This subfile also claims that physical inactivity is harmful to general metabolic health, which may be due to the damage it causes to the ability of tissues to metabolize both fatty acids and sugar. The electronic literature also discusses the potential health-enhancing benefits that stem from physical activity, including a reduction in heart rate and resistance to the accumulation of heart disease in general. More than 60 minutes of physical activity accumulation each day was found to act as a significant driver of heart health improvement. Studies have found that extracurricular activities actually help to increase basal metabolism and increase energy acceptance for the 24-hour day/night cycle.

All search results of the various databases are saved in a Microsoft Word file. This main file is divided into subfiles on different categories of causes of bladder cancer in females. For example, there is a subfile labeled 6.3 Physical Inactivity that is a potential cause of bladder cancer in females. Each of these subfiles includes electronic literature (words of text) related to the specific cause that is labeled as our official hypotheses. All of this information was written by Ramakrishnan S., a collaborator who sometimes helps to organize these files after downloading them from the various electronic databases.

7. Environmental Carcinogens

Occupation Historically, workplace exposure to certain naturally-occurring chemicals, such as those used in dyeing, rubber production, and aluminum processing, were associated with the development of bladder cancer. Although safety controls have since been put in place in the industrialized world, there is still a risk of workplace exposure in other parts of the world. In addition to industrial chemicals, workers who are occupationally exposed to carcinogens such as metals or solvents may be at increased risk of developing bladder cancer. Working with these substances is associated with an increased risk of developing bladder cancer. In men who work with such substances, workplace exposure has been linked to the development of bladder cancer. Overall, though, industrial hygiene has improved and the number of workplace exposures has decreased with the onset of sustainably-manufactured synthetic materials. In women who work in exposed workplaces, such as hairdressers, no clear association has been demonstrated.

Risk Factors for Bladder Cancer Exposures to potential cancer-causing agents, either in the workplace or through lifestyle habits, have been linked to the majority of bladder cancers.

The onset of the disease is also affected by the environment, where several environmental factors, including environmental toxins and occupational carcinogens, are associated with a different risk of developing bladder cancer. The frequency of contamination and exposure is the primary reason for the higher incidence in specific areas of the world.

6. Explaining Bladder Cancer in Females

8. Medical Conditions and Treatments Associated with Bladder Cancer

Introduction Certain medical conditions such as pelvic irradiation, neurogenic bladder, end-stage renal failure, selected chronic infections, and recurrent urinary tract infections, and specific types of medications have been associated with the occurrence of bladder cancer. Identification of potential risk factors gives an option for inflammation as it might contribute to the development and progression of malignancy. Since the potential occurrence of bladder carcinoma-in-situ was a possible reason to justify transurethral bladder biopsies, doing so in patients with side effects of high-dose prophylaxis became a priority. This study had a broad-based inclusion strategy and an extensive anti-tumor prophylaxis list, including calcium phosphate for some of them. There is evidence that specific treatments, such as working in a solvent-exposed environment, might improve patient results. The adjustment of medication use to affect gene code expression of tumor was also an objective of the review. Specific agents that are involved include diethylstilbestrol, telomerase inhibitors, cyclophosphamide, halogenated agents, and others. Tumor makeup can affect bladder cancer, such as populations that comprise people with spinal cord injuries who are most susceptible to bladder malignancy. The existence of a congenital urinary bladder problematic is notated as grade Hin lampatta te ra. It is well known that fewer women are written than men, but behavioral adjustment and tobacco threat are blamed for the primary result.

Bladder cancer is a multifactorial disease. The etiology of spontaneous urinary bladder cancer is heterogeneous, with various genetic, environmental, occupational, lifestyle, and medical factors that could increase individuals' susceptibility to the disease. There is a growing body of evidence showing associations or potential associations between certain medical conditions and treatments and risk or prognosis of bladder carcinoma in situ (CIS), muscle-invasive, and non-muscle-invasive bladder cancer (NMIBC).

8.1. Bladder Birth Defects

It is possible but not well-proven that urinary bladder birth defects cause cancer in females. Bladder birth defects are very uncommon in females. Some genital birth defects may be connected with renal birth defects. Benign kidney swelling after puberty can be caused by a uterine tumor that blocks urine flow (vaginal septate plate). Women may also have double chambered bladders, and this condition would be asked during physical examination. Many individuals are having long-term side effects following cancer diagnosis and treatment as a result of their diagnosis and treatment; these problems often increase as the length of time since the original treatment increases.

Female-specific bladder cancers, such as bladder exstrophy squamous metaplasia carcinoma and cloacal exstrophy adenocarcinoma, have been associated with other congenital genitourinary anomalies like Mayer-Rokitansky-Küster-Hauser (MRKH) syndrome, which does raise suspicion for the inherent connection between genitourinary birth defects and cancer of those tissues. If the way that an individual forms is wrong, there may be a problem with the tissue that those cells create. This is one of the things that we have to watch for long term when you see an individual who may have been born with abnormal tissues based on the conditions listed below.

8.2. Bladder Infections and Stones

Urinary stones may form in the kidneys, ureters, or urinary bladder, and may increase the risk of bladder cancer. Some stones grow bacteria, which could release extra carcinogenic compounds into the bladder. Stones can famously form around small beads or foreign material that gets stuck in the bladder. In 2006, the International Agency for Research on Cancer concluded that there was inadequate evidence in humans for the carcinogenicity of "foci of squamous cell tumors as a consequence of foreign bodies, infection, calculus or Hanssen-Flemming disease, in the urinary bladder of females." Urinary stones might reflect both infection and lifestyle trends that can also increase risk. For example, American women with stones are significantly more likely to have had a hysterectomy or treatment for urinary incontinence than women without stones. A recent American study showed a significant 40% increase in the risk of bladder cancer for women who have had hysterectomies. Chronic infection and inflammation, presumably largely in women, emerges as the outstanding long-term determinant of environmental and occupational exposures to bladder cancer.

The existence of bladder infection alone has not yielded a consistent association with bladder cancer. The causative agents of urinary tract infections (or bladder infections) have been found in the urinary bladder of up to 65% of females with acute symptoms, and up to 99% of females with chronic symptoms. Between recurring episodes, the bladder may accumulate a layer of infected biofilm, often showing few symptoms. It has also been established that the lack of symptoms, called asymptomatic bacteriuria, is both common and may result in chronic infection. Given that most urinary tract infections occur within only 2-3 years of a previous urinary tract infection, it is important to study the effects, if any, of such frequent infections.

9. Conclusion and Future Research Directions

Future research should be focused on the macrosocial aspects related to women's breast cancer health, especially regarding procedures for reducing breast cancer occurrence in younger generations, similarly deepening, in addition to the etiological aspects of that matter, a more accurate evaluation of women at risk and preventive medical examinations. Many areas remain to be explored. For example, just to mention a few, a study on urinary metabolites in relation to the menstrual cycle, although postulated, is still missing, as is a study comparing the urinary metabolic and hormonal changes of women who have undergone a hysterectomy and not necessarily experienced natural menopause with the castrate ones. In terms of the metabolic and genetic approach, work is also lacking about comparing the metabolome and expression analysis of breast cancer, at different stages of female life, with that of male breast cancer. Any further information will help to clarify whether discrimination, and to what extent, should be included in the ongoing studies.

Currently, there is no evident research on female breast cancer shared depending on the same study subjects like age and gender. This limits well-founded conclusions, since the breast cancer evolution in females can be multi-etiological, predicated upon the said interactions. This lack of evidence may also be the cause of the variously specified causative risk factors in the reviews and meta-analyses.

Then, more biological or clinical mediators can explain the causal relationships, especially related to the emotional and the menopausal changes in life. Therefore, at present, the limited comparison between the various gender results does not provide great elements of novelty, instead quite a lot of confirmations; rather, it raises future insights in female health theories formation.

Potential Causes and Early Signs of Bladder Cancer in Females

1. Introduction to Bladder Cancer in Females

The possible differences in the appearance of urinary bladder cancer in females stimulated an interest in clarifying potential differences in the pathogenesis and development of this malignancy. The research reports an analysis of selected references following a search performed in June 2021 on Medline/PubMed in English to explore potential risk factors and early clinical signs and symptoms of bladder cancer, particularly in females. Full paper records concerning both pathogenesis and etiological agents of bladder cancer and the symptoms of this neoplasm in females and males were included. Data from multicenter or national single-center, large-scale research and consensus reports based on systematic literature searches were preferred. The main exclusion criteria were: papers not related to the analyzed clinical questions, research by non-oncological or genitourinary oncological teams, and reviews.

However, a large variety of these regional risk factors such as urinary and schistosomal infections are not common etiological agents in the developed part of Europe and the USA. Possible additional causes of bladder cancer which may be related to alterations in the urothelial exposition to potentially harmful compounds, like different patterns and urine concentrations of carcinogenic metabolites or proteomic differences - a cluster of biomarkers.

The pathogenesis of bladder cancer seems to be multifactorial as it involves several established and potential etiological agents. Repeated irritation of the bladder urothelium with phenacetin, with concomitant use of non-steroidal anti-inflammatory compounds, infections, schistosomiasis, inappropriate hygiene, smoking, artificial sweeteners, ionizing radiation, and potential occupational and drug exposure may contribute to carcinogenesis of the urinary bladder.

Bladder cancer is one of the most commonly diagnosed malignancies with relatively high morbidity and mortality frequencies worldwide, and the number of new cases per year is still growing. According to available data, males are approximately four times more commonly affected by bladder cancer than females. Nevertheless, statistics from the American Cancer Society showed that the morbidity rate becomes similar with age, and after the age of 85 years, the risk of developing this disease in females becomes even higher.

2. Epidemiology of Bladder Cancer in Females

In general, the average age at diagnosis for bladder cancer is 73 years, and the age-standardized rate is approximately sevenfold higher for men than for women. While the race with the highest incidence of bladder cancer is white, followed by an Asian population, the race that consumes the least amount of alcohol is African American. In parallel to this, bladder cancer is seen in white and Asian cases before African American races. Residential history has been shown to exhibit an increase in bladder cancer. Erol et al. have found that while individuals living in high-arsenic and heavy metal-contaminated areas are five times more likely to succumb to bladder cancer than the U.S. general population, the prevalence of bladder cancer in patients living in areas contaminated with arsenic/heavy metals was statistically significantly higher.

Bladder cancer predominates in men, among whom men are 3-4 times more likely to succumb to the disease than females. The reason for this male prevalence is related to lifestyle factors, occupational exposures, and anatomical differences from urinary systems. As a result, unlike prostate cancer, it is difficult to measure the exact incidence and prevalence and to investigate the genetic aspects of carcinoma arising in women's bladder. Studies have shown that, as with carcinoma, the incidence of bladder cancer increases in females starting from the age of 55 years. According to the 2020 National Cancer

Institute statistics, it is seen that while the prevalence and incidence of bladder cancer in males is around 45,000 and 147,000, these values decrease to about 17,500 and 44,100 in women. This means that the incidence of individuals with bladder cancer among females is about 31.7 per 100,000.

3. Risk Factors for Bladder Cancer in Females

1. Smoking: While this is the topmost cause for developing cancer of the bladder in both males and females, smoking is more common in females compared to males. It has also been found to be more harmful, with females being at an increased risk of developing bladder cancer for a longer duration compared to men who smoke. The risk is relatively high among women who have been heavy smokers. 2. Misusing Tobacco: Female bladder cancer patients have often developed the disease after using tobacco products such as chewing tobacco, snuff, and dipping tobacco for many years. 3. Chronic Bladder Infections: In women, those with chronic bladder infections or inflammation (cystitis) have a higher likelihood of developing bladder cancer. 4. Long-term Catheter Use: Due to advanced age or other causes, some women require a tube with a bag to drain urine (catheter) for several years. Long-term use of these catheters has been found to be a potential cause of developing squamous cell cancer of the bladder, even though it's relatively rare compared to other bladder cancer types.

Bladder cancer is known to be more common in women than in men. According to the American Cancer Society, about 36,000 women and 83,000 men are diagnosed with the disease each year. Though it may sound alarming, there are several potential risk factors that are known for the development of bladder cancer in females, with smoking or having smoked in the past being the topmost cause. What's more, a detailed understanding of these risk factors can help us find the potential causes of cancer and tips for an early diagnosis, which are yet to be known.

3.1. Smoking

In contrast, the early events involved in tumor development in smokers are still poorly understood. Reviews of the literature often describe these superoxide dismutase events in smokers as a "protective effect," given the antioxidant effect of this enzyme. However, it is clear from recent in vitro studies that the female membrane pattern "only" could have a high antioxidant rate because of a composition in unsaturated fatty acids. The protective effect of coffee consumption is also another controversial issue with gender.

This hypothesis is supported by in vitro studies where female smokers presented a 30% increased risk of bladder cancer compared to non-smokers, a probability specific to this gender. This induces tumor initiation or tumor progression for those who develop a hyperactive pattern of the superoxide dismutase enzyme (SOD) as an antioxidant response specific to early events in tumor development and seen in exposed female smokers.

Bladder cancer is a multifactorial disease, with smoking being the key risk factor in the development of this disease in women. Epidemiological studies confirm the strong association of smoking with the initiation and progression of bladder tumors, as well as their recurrence. Tobacco chemicals are typically metabolized into reactive intermediates that cause mutations and/or genomic instability because the host's detoxification mechanisms are ineffective or limited.

3.2. Chemical Exposure

The main identified risk factor is cigarette smoking, as the risk of any form of cancer increases in response to tobacco smoke containing known carcinogens, such as heterocyclic amines, which are suspected to increase risk via a nitrosamine travelling the bloodstream to the bladder. Kaplan et al.'s review of literature discovered a non-significant increase for the risks for workers, in fact, the SIR for commercial-worker (14.0) is marginally higher than that for manufacturer-worker cancer morbidity (13.4) which is supported by Pelissero and Riding, considering the UK dyestuff worker SIR's were 15.4 (1980s) and 43.5 (1940s). In 1950, Niedham and Conston pre-empted the cancer of the bladder morbidity for the United States, with over 220,000 women workers being exposed to commercial and manufacturer dyes. Therefore, they expected an extra rate of 10-20 ness including bladder cancer. Jurjus, in 2004, discussed what happened to women who, after World War II, were employed in the shoe industry until 1965. The exposure to the same dyes (benzidine or direct dyes) as the men that were in their workplace produced a significant increase in deaths from cancers, including bladder cancer. Other studies have shown that women who smoke may almost double their chances of dying from bladder cancer if they come into contact with chemicals like benzene. In fact, new studies show that while only about 1 in 73 women in the general population will develop cancer of the twisting tubes in their lifetime, among women show drivers (low level of benzene) 1 in 20 will. Chromosomal damage involving proto-oncogene activation has been seen in 54% of female dyers who are smokers and in 50% of female dyers who worked with the industry within the prior year.

Cigarette Smoking

Some studies have reported a correlation between chemical exposure and an augmented inclination to develop bladder cancer in women when compared to women who do not undergo chemical exposure. Schulte et al. state that women who work in the textile or fabric printing industry are particularly vulnerable to bladder cancer due to azo and 4-aminobiphenyl exposure, although they are also exposed to formaldehyde and phenol which have been described as having an estrogen-like impact. Women who work with dyes and pigments are becoming increasingly engaged in some specific job functions associated with a significant rise in the risk of bladder neoplasia. For many dye stuffs including diaminotoluenes and benzidines, where there is sufficient data available, formaldehyde (present in dyestuff formulations) seemed to have estrogenic effects thereby increasing the likelihood of breast and uterine cancer. Dye preparation and operation bench handlings are positive relative risk three compared to disease morbidity cross genders. Formaldehyde is widely used in histological and laboratory preparation where a two-fold increase in breast cancer has been reported in women who work in this industry. Schulte et al. describe other substances obtainable work-related sources used in industries dominated by women, which have adverse effects on the bladder. For example, in the shoe industry, formaldehyde is utilized in shoe development glues where a significant increased risk of bladder neoplasia is evident in a Canadian study of 1700 dyer and processor operatives. Furthermore, the pretanning practice of women hide workers involves mining lime and dolomite deposit where a variety of jobs exposing the worker to dust (e.g., laboring) would place the employer at increased susceptibility to mines that have asbestos. A two-fold increase in bladder neoplasia has been noted with the pretanning industry.

4. Pathophysiology of Bladder Cancer in Females

Bladder cancer is mainly caused by the combined action of exogenous environment and endogenous tissue, which triggers and stimulates the chronic injury repair sequence of the bladder epithelium. The initial cause of bladder cancer is mainly related to smoking, chemical dyes, or industrial pollutants due to inflammation, genetic mutations of bladder cells, and development of three stages: initiation, promotion, and progressive development of bladder carcinogenesis. According to the increased membrane permeability and the leaked soluble urine carcinogens to the submucosal region to absorb, these irreversible cumulative DNA mutations included meeting with proto-oncogene and tumor suppressor gene (TSG) two major types. In recent years, with the further development of molecular biology and protein chip in the early screening of bladder cancer, found that the up-regulated urinary excretion could benefit the early diagnosis of bladder cancer. Early prevention of causes and predisposing signs of bladder cancer in women needs longitudinal and in-depth studies to explore, which provides theoretical guidance for clinical prevention, early diagnosis, and timely treatment of bladder cancer in women.

Bladder cancer is the major malignant tumor of the urinary system that is associated with high morbidity and mortality. Over 400,000 new cases are reported each year.

Among these tumors, transitional cell carcinoma accounts for over 90% of cases. Considering the role innate biological differences and carcinogen exposure play in producing bladder cancer, the degree of molecular genetic alterations of tumor cells, as well as the surrounding normal tissue, can provide a comprehensive view of cancer development. Although molecular genetics is developing rapidly, no major advances have been reported in the areas of tumor suppressor genes, oncogenes, DNA repair gene alterations, or biologically significant alterations involved in hormonal effects. Painless hematuria is the most important early symptom of bladder cancer. Therefore, any woman with unexplained hematuria should be referred for an appropriate evaluation for potential underlying malignancies such as bladder cancer or urinary tract infection. This paper presents reports indicating the early signs of females with bladder cancer, especially mild or chronic symptoms that were previously ignored. Exploring these changes could provide guidance in effective prevention, early diagnosis, and timely treatment of bladder cancer.

5. Clinical Presentation of Bladder Cancer in Females

Early signs of bladder cancer: Hematuria can serve as an introduction to bladder cancer. It can be of either macroscopic or microscopic character or with potential recurrence. Macroscopic hematuria can be easily recognized by patients. Microscopic hematuria is three times as frequent among patients diagnosed with bladder cancer and has an 8-18-fold increase in the risk of malignancy compared to untreated patients. Early signs and symptoms: The most accepted early clinical manifestations of bladder cancer are hematuria and morbidity of unknown causes. Hematuria is reported in 40-80% of all adult patients eventually diagnosed with bladder cancer; the majority have episodes of visible (macroscopic or microscopic) hematuria.

Clinical presentation of bladder cancer in females: Hematuria is still the most common presenting complaint of urinary malignancy, ultimately prompting investigation. Until recently, its presence had not been positively correlated with the diagnosis of bladder cancer. The authors' trust, and studies that have been reviewed lately excluded gender examination, which is pivotal in including investigated patients. Infringing these studies, along with the early research work of Restriction with Bladder Cancer and Single Serum alarms, all found warnings of existence in higher instances of macroscopic or dipseroscopic irregularities in the organ, especially nodular-looking ones.

5.1. Early Signs

For this reason, it is important that professionals responsible for diagnosing the disease trim the possible causes with all possible advances and have an even more objective diagnosis, through the results obtained in more detailed diagnostic tests. Detailed knowledge on the signs and symptoms of BC are essential for an earlier detection of the disease, improving the patient's chances of a cure. A recent review involving 351 biopsies from patients with irritative symptoms suggested a high diagnostic rate, leading to the authors to conclude that in selected patients, irritative symptoms could be interpreted as flashlights pointing towards early-stage bladder cancer. Hematuria is detection simply evaluate if patient attributes it has color or not.

This study is Section 5: Potential Causes and Early Signs of Bladder Cancer in Females. Objective: This chapter provides a comprehensive overview of potential causes and early signs of bladder cancer. Specifically centering on the early signs of bladder cancer in females, demonstrated that these signs include, but are not limited to, hematuria, pollakiuria, urgency, and dysuria. The experts agreed that the initial diagnostic methods should involve a physical examination and patient history, such as whether or not the patient has a family medical history of bladder cancer; other potential causes, such as urinary tract infections or other bladder conditions; and toxic work environments or exposure to potential carcinogens. Subjective complaints, such as pollakiuria, urgency, and dysuria, are also flashing signs of early-stage disease. pointed out that with the collection of a precise anamnesis, it is possible to suggest that the prevalence of any concomitant potential causes does not necessarily influence the risk of developing bladder cancer, since about 60% of new bladder cancer diagnoses are not related to typical risk factors or causes.

5.2. Symptoms in Advanced Stages

Most of the initially emerging bladder cancer symptoms might be connected to urination. They incorporate pain during urination, which is medically termed as dysuria, a condition that might arise from the tumor promptly intervening with the open flow of the urine outwardly from an affected bladder. Bladder cancer might also trigger one's need to urinate more often than typical, which is termed polyuria, and may necessitate night-time urination, a condition known as nocturia. Micturition signifies the act of urinating and presented this light, haematuria—hence bladder cancer—could be apparent when one is trying to pee. As the disorder gets worse, the symptoms could extend into one's body. One might also observe anguish about the bladder, known as suprapubic crusade. The physical manifestation might signal that the tumor has begun to surpass the bladder layer, and pressure instigates the discomfort.

Haematuria, or the appearance of blood in one's urine, is the predominant precise clinical indication of bladder cancer at any phase. Though the majority of bladder tumors are classified as non-malignant clutters, females who acquire bladder cancer display similar initial clinical indications to males, offering haematuria as the key or one of the indistinguishable clinical symptoms. Also, they convey a greater bladder cancer analysis occurrence. This might be linked to the fact that differential analyzing or verification protocols have coupled modalities for females and males, leading females matching analytical and research chances when both genders emerged as a single populace in datasets. Thus, attempts must be applied towards bridging the gender analytical breach that may eventually aid in dealing with bladder cancer more effectively.

6. Diagnostic Approaches for Bladder Cancer in Females

The majority of women with bladder cancer have non-muscle-invasive tumors at diagnosis. These require a transurethral resection of the bladder tumor (TURBT) to remove them, which is also used to stage the depth of invasion of the tumor. If susceptible features of bladder cancer are recognized in the TURBT specimens, then patients are given intravesical BCG to melt away any residual disease and may also be offered adjuvant chemotherapy. In the literature, it is reported that the average length of the delay of bladder cancer diagnosis caused by the misdiagnosis as UTI ranges from 0 to 30 months in females. Although the ultrasound might contribute to the diagnosis of bladder disorders, it is stated that cystoscopy or having a urine cytology test must not be delayed. The diagnosis of women with a history of recurrent UTI must also include bladder cancer, and this possibility must not arise.

Available evidence suggests that the diagnosis of bladder cancer in females is a clinical challenge, as the symptoms suggesting bladder cancer are common and seen usually due to benign infections and conditions. Here, imaging techniques, including contrast-enhanced computed tomography (CT), are essential for the diagnosis of urinary tract obstruction, environment of the bladder, and upper urinary tract tumors. As the preoperative rate of deep muscle invasive bladder cancer on TURBT is disappointingly low (7-61% in recent series), various imaging techniques are increasingly utilized to stage bladder tumors invasively, psychologically and pathologically. Cystoscopy, which has 61% sensitivity but 95% specificity, is taken as the diagnostic gold standard for identification of the bladder tumor. Several cystoscopy procedures such as liquid-based cytology or image enhancement can also be used for early bladder tumor detection.

6.1. Imaging Techniques

For patients with breast cancer, cross-sectional imaging can offer detailed information of the extent of disease. Post-resection, cross-sectional imaging can detect residual masses and evaluate response to treatment. Furthermore, some imaging findings are independent predictors of patient outcomes and help guide management. The typical imaging findings of breast cancer, disease susceptibility by location, and lesion characteristics on CT, MR, and ultrasonography are summarized in Table 6. Magnetic resonance imaging during the initial evaluation can provide detailed information on the whole picture of the disease extension of breast carcinoma, which is necessary for the use of appropriate treatment modalities. In case of patients with muscle-invasive cancer on MR, DWI and T2-weighted imaging can be used for detecting metastases to local lymph nodes. Ultrasonography can be used for the initial approach to detect simple breast tumors and can be used as part of a scheme (triphasic cystosonography) to detect the invasion of the detrusor muscle.

Imaging in the evaluation of breast cancer in females can be done using various imaging modalities listed in 6.1.1. MR imaging has evolved for staging and assessing disease response in breast cancer, with distinct advantages in low-risk and high-risk non-muscle invasive breast cancer due to its superior ability to depict the depth of tumor invasion and differentiation between low-grade and high-grade tumor. Furthermore, MR imaging has been shown to have clinical utility in detecting breast cancer recurrences and pathological staging as compared to clinical evaluation. CT, especially for initial imaging, is contrast-enhanced but it has low sensitivity for T-stage disease and recurrence compared to MR imaging. Additionally, FDG-PET for bladder cancer remains investigational, and in comparison to MR, FDG-PET offers limited soft tissue detail without a clear dichotomy on breast cancer aggressiveness. Ultrasound of the bladder is generally insensitive compared to CT and MR; however, triphasic ultrasound cystosonography shows potential in diagnosing the depth of invasion of breast cancer lesions.

6.2. Biopsy

Transurethral resection of bladder tumor: This is also called TURBT or TUR. During this surgical procedure, a needle-like tool called a resectoscope is inserted into the body via the urethra. The resectoscope enables the healthcare provider to both visualize and remove part or all of a tumor with an attached wire loop. Through this wire, an electrical current burns the tumor away and cuts the tissue or tumor from the bladder wall. The removed part is then examined under a microscope to determine the extent of the tumor's spread and type. It also assists in determining if and where it has spread and can help the healthcare provider estimate whether and where it is likely to come back. Typically, the results of the biopsy come back around one week to ten days later. The pathologist, a doctor who specializes in diagnosing diseases by examining tissue and cells under a microscope, writes a report on what they find. The results of your biopsy can confirm if you do have bladder cancer, as well as provide information on the type and grade (how aggressive the cancer is). It's only after diagnosis that your healthcare provider will be able to recommend the best types of treatment and advice for you.

If you have symptoms, such as red urine or a lesion in your bladder discovered during imaging or cystoscopy, your healthcare provider may recommend that you undergo a procedure called a biopsy. There are a few different tools to collect tissue for a biopsy: a transurethral resection of bladder tumor (TURBT), an endoscopic biopsy, or a miniMAG.

7. Treatment Modalities for Bladder Cancer in Females

Several drugs continue to be prescribed by urological oncologists. The exact choice of drug is based on several factors, including the muscle-invasive status of the cancer, any markers of response and whether it is treatment-naïve or a second or later line of treatment. There are three main classes of drugs that treat muscle-invasive, metastatic or recurrent cancer of the bladder. Surgery: Radical cystectomy is commonly performed in females as men. The surgeon can create a new bladder for holding urine. If the affected individual's bladder has been removed, urine may exit through a hole in the skin of the abdomen, called a stoma, and be collected in a bag outside the body. Preliminary study also suggests that cystectomy can also reduce the risk of dying from bladder cancer in females. Chemotherapy: One mode of decreasing the risk of recurrence is the use of intravesical chemotherapy in high-risk non-invasive disease. The usual regime is weekly MMC for six weeks with further instillation at 3 months and then six monthly or 3 monthly thereafter for a further year. In some females, instillation of BCG (intravesical immunotherapy) is used to reduce the risk of recurrence.

Bladder cancer in females can be managed in a number of ways. These include endoscopic resection of the tumor, repeat surveillance of the tumor at regular intervals with cystoscopy and urine cytology, intravesical chemotherapy, intravesical immunotherapy, and progression to radical cystectomy. Cystectomy in general was found to be associated with a significantly lower risk of death than an endoscopic approach in females with non-muscle invasive cancer. In a study by Stein et al., the trend reversed in a small subset of female patients who had high grade, muscle-invasive cancer. Complete or partial cystectomy is the standard therapy for muscle-invasive bladder cancer. However, radical cystectomy is a complex surgery with relatively high rates of postoperative complications and perioperative mortality.

7.1. Surgery

Indeed, the most common treatment is the removal of the body of the bladder, with up to 60% of bladder surgery performed in males over 65 and up to 48% in women of the same age. However, the surgical management of tumors of the bladder in elderly women and children has limited applicability. Patients treated with local BCG (bacillus Calmette-Guerin) are among the most frequent populations that require bladder removal. Regionally significant patients are followed by external beam therapy combined with concomitant chemotherapy. However, radio-chemotherapy for bladder preserving treatments requires long resting hospitalization, and there is also an increased length of greater than 60 months of age. Radical cystectomy (RE) forms the basic treatment option for muscle-invasive bladder cancer (MIBC) in females. Polychemotherapy (PCH) with methotrexate, vinblastine, doxorubicin and cisplatinum (MVAC) and adjuvant chemotherapy improves the survival of patients. A urinary stoma, compared with nil in normal subjects, can have a negative effect on the quality of life of some individuals and requires revision within 10 years of construction. Other alternative surgical procedures like the retubularized ureteric re-implantation in the bowel have a shorter stenosis-free time when compared to the non-evacuating urinary conduit. However, neobladder performed well with no evidence of re-obstruction on long term follow up. On the other hand, neobladder recovery, and a short hospital stay, are compromised by longer catheterization. Various surgical interventions are also indicated for the treatment of long-term complications of major surgery. Often, bladder mucosal reconstruction should solve the problem after inadvertent mucosal ice. After successful initial management of cancer of the bladder, lifelong annual cystoscopy is advised. Post-radiation urinary fistula with the rectum is another rare but serious side effect which establishes communication between the bladder and rectum. This brief communication is intended to discuss possible causes and early symptoms of female bladder carcinoma.

Bladder cancer in females, although relatively rare in comparison to their male counterparts, is definitely a pressing health issue. The primary course of treatment is surgery. Surgery can be undertaken by various methods (both traditional and minimally invasive); some procedures may require complete removal of the bladder. Surgery can also be combined, if necessary, with radiation therapy and chemotherapy. Following such procedures, various surgical (urinary stoma) and non-surgical (ureterostomy cutis, main intra-articular drainage, orthotopic ileal neo-bladder, penile urethra, and vesicovaginal fistula creation) interventions are available for continuity treatment. Several methods such as bladder mucosal freezing, perfusion chemotherapy, hyperbaric oxygen therapy, and urine excretion can also be effectively used to alleviate their complications. Bladder cancer in females, which is the eighth largest health problem for women in the British Isles behind ovarian cancer, causes an average of 30 deaths annually. It is seen primarily in post-menopausal females aged between 60 and 69 who have given birth to two or three children. Treatment of this condition so far has been mainly focused on surgery and follows a detailed flow chart as shown in Figure 1.

7.2. Chemotherapy

For many years, there is no systemic treatment in patients with advanced bladder cancer who have received surgery of the tumor and established carcinoma, who have signs of the disease, and a tumor is detected in another organ in all patients who have received surgery with a cystectomy. Chemotherapy has been shown to increase the cystectomy area, although the number of systemic diseases that have been started has been increased. However, the progressive improvement of chemotherapy agents in the last 20 years has allowed the disease to be controlled in women with advanced-stage illness. The substances used are called platinum derivatives (cisplatin and carboplatin) except for some exceptions, and these drugs are applied alone or in combination with other appropriate drugs. The principle of chemotherapy is that, by reaching every cell in the body, all of the cells, cancerous and healthy, are affected by the drug, and especially cancer cells are more affected than healthy ones and prevent the growth of existing cells.

Bladder cancer is a disease in which abnormal cell growth occurs in the urinary system and mainly affects females. This may start from hormone changes, long-term exposure to toxic substances, as well as smoking, which fertilizes waste products. However, it is not specific to these causes, and a definite cause cannot be interpreted. As the tumor is arranged, the characteristics of the tissue invaded by the bladder wall, and whether it affects the neighboring lymph nodes (M) or distant organs, the determination of the treatment options is made. The first treatment is often extensive surgical excision and removal of the bladder, and in order to prevent metastasis, removal of nearby lymph nodes is performed.

7.3. Immunotherapy

Immunotherapies (also called immune-based strategies, therapies, or agents; corruption of the immune system) are treatments that use the body's natural defenses or its design to fight infection or different diseases. Experimental immunotherapies that are currently being tested as a treatment for bladder cancer stimulate the body to make the immune cells that help the patient's body attack the cancer by increasing the strength of the immune system by helping the immune system to better its job as boosting the ability to get rid of cancer. When the body can't get rid of symptoms, immunotherapy can sometimes help. Immunotherapy can help the body better see cancer by a woman's body to try to get cancer and keep it under control. More recently, scientists have developed altogether immune cells known as T-cells to go and kill cancer cells. T-cells will regenerate to bound worn-out white blood cells and keep a trace of specifically that changed them to turn protection on. By creating a cell that uses T-cells to significantly kill the cancerous cells, we can even get the human system to assault the cancer.

As the immunotherapeutic approach is about optimizing the patient's own immune defense reactions to help him oppose the tumor, this treatment modality has attracted considerable interest and following in clinical research in the last decade, not only as a supplement but also as an alternative treatment method in common clinical practice for many tumors. This mini review focuses on novel information from immunotherapy approaches and the use of this treatment strategy exclusively on FBC in females.

Immunotherapy as a new treatment modality in bladder cancer in females

8. Prognosis and Survival Rates in Females with Bladder Cancer

• The 5-year survival rate for cancer that has not spread beyond the inner lining layer of the bladder is about 70%. • The 5-year survival rate for cancer that has invaded the lamina propria connective tissue layer of the bladder is about 65%. • The 5-year survival rate for cancer that has invaded the thick muscle wall of the bladder is about 20%. • The 5-year survival rate for cancer that has extended through the bladder wall and invade surrounding structures such as the prostate, ovary, uterus, or vagina and for cancer that has spread to lymph nodes in the pelvis is about 5%.

The 5-year relative survival rates based on the stage of the cancer are as follows:

• The stage of the cancer at the time of diagnosis • Tumor grade • Is there more than one tumor in the bladder? • Size and number of tumors • The response to treatment • Age • Overall health • Type of bladder cancer • Any long-term effects from the cancer or treatment.

Prognosis refers to the process of determining the expected outcome of an individual's disease, including the effect of the disease on the individual's quality of life. For individuals with bladder cancer, prognosis is determined by the following clinical and demographic factors:

Prognosis and Survival Rates in Females

Bladder Cancer

9. Preventive Strategies for Bladder Cancer in Females

Measures are often needed to protect women. Early signs of bleeding from the bladder, a change in bladder habits including frequent urination, pain or urgency during urination, recurring urinary tract infections, and general discomfort in the pelvic area and back should not be neglected. In the event of these early signs, individuals are advised to visit their doctor for testing. In order to control the quality of life and reduce the incidence, it is wise to change protective or modifying lifestyle factors that are associated with the emergence of bladder cancer, such as quitting smoking and reducing exposure to chemicals in industry. Regular consultation with the society, which can screen people with dysuria, urinary bleeding, or urinary abnormalities to determine the incidence, located in early signs of female's bladder cancer.

Studies have reported a gradual rise in the number of bladder cancer cases in female individuals in the past few decades. Identifying the potential causes and early signs of bladder cancer in females could pave the way to develop a cure for this type of cancer. Certain measures can be very useful tools in the fight to reduce the likelihood of developing this dysfunctional disease. Such measures include the intake of more fluids, moderate physical activity, physical examinations, regular use of cranberry supplements, and proper living habits. The purpose of this paper is to use library-based research to shed light on some preventive strategies that can be effective in preventing a variety of bladder cancers in females. Given that the development of all types of bladder cancers is usually associated with potential risk factors, these preventive strategies could mitigate the potential causes of bladder cancer in female individuals.

www.ingramcontent.com/pod-product-compliance
Lightning Source LLC
Chambersburg PA
CBHW050850260726
48660CB00006B/2542